HOMEMADE
Nail Polish

HOMEMADE
Nail Polish

Create Unique Colors and Designs
for Stunning Nails

ALLISON ROSE
SPIEKERMANN

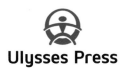

Ulysses Press

Published in the U.S. by
Ulysses Press
P.O. Box 3440
Berkeley, CA 94703
www.ulyssespress.com

ISBN: 978-1-61243-307-3
Library of Congress Control Number 2013957315

Printed in the United States by Bang Printing

10 9 8 7 6 5 4 3 2 1

Acquisitions Editor: Kelly Reed
Managing Editor: Claire Chun
Editor: Kate St. Clair
Proofreader: Barbara Schultz
Cover design: Michelle Thompson
Interior design and layout: what!design @ whatweb.com
Cover photographs: front © Meera Lee Patel; back © Allison Rose Spiekermann

Distributed by Publishers Group West

IMPORTANT NOTE TO READERS: This book is independently authored and published and no sponsorship or endorsement of this book by, and no affiliation with, any trademarked brands or other products mentioned or pictured within is claimed or suggested. All trademarks that appear in directions, photographs, and elsewhere in this book belong to their respective owners and are used here for informational purposes only. The author and publishers encourage readers to patronize the quality brands and products mentioned and pictured in this book.

To Max, for everything

Table of Contents

Introduction

Wearing nail polish is a fast, fun, and easy way to express your creativity through color and design. But have you ever been inspired to wear a color that just "didn't exist"? Or wanted to create a polish inspired by a picture you've seen or to match an outfit for a special occasion?

This book is designed to teach anyone to be able to mix unique nail polish colors quickly, easily, and consistently—and often using nothing more than what is available at your local drug store. A detailed section on equipment and ingredients will explain what each item can be used for and its benefits to you as you begin your mixing adventure.

Interested in glittery polishes? Learn about the different colors, sizes, shapes, and finishes of glitter—and which are best suited for use in polish. Have you tried mixing polish but ended up with separated or lumpy polish? I've also included techniques that will help you improve existing polishes using a combination of mixing and application techniques.

By following the more than 30 recipes provided here, you will become familiar with the concepts of mixing colors—even adding special-effects pigments to make your creations really stand out. Along the way there are photos and instructions to guide you and, ultimately, prepare you to begin mixing your own unique color combinations!

Finally, there are chapters that cover nail polish application and nail art techniques so you can best showcase your handmade polishes.

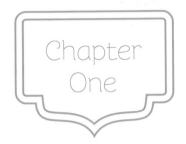

Chapter
One

Ingredients:
What They Are, What They Do,
and What to Look For

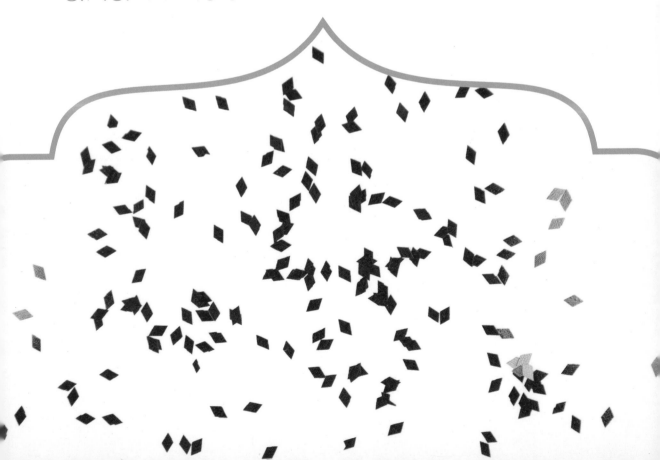

Before you begin making your own nail polish, it's helpful to understand what the main ingredients are and what they do. All nail polish begins with basically three types of ingredients: film-forming agents, plasticizers, and solvents. Different manufacturers will use various ratios of these ingredients (a closely guarded secret!) in an effort to optimize wear, application, and appearance.

The main ingredients, the ones usually listed first, are solvents. These are what help keep the polish a workable consistency that can be applied to the nail neatly. A combination of quicker- and slower-evaporating solvents are used so that immediately after application, the quicker-evaporating solvents help set the polish, but the slower-evaporating solvents allow the polish to level, which eliminates brushstrokes and creates a smooth finish. Ethyl acetate and butyl acetate are the most popular solvents, having replaced toluene in today's 3-free formulations. Somewhat recently (beginning in the early 2000's) there was a move by nail polish companies to eliminate toluene, formaldehyde, and dibutyl phthalate from their formulations due to actions taken by the European Union to limit or ban these ingredients in cosmetics. Today most nail polishes available are advertised as "three-free" or "3-free" which refers to the fact that they don't contain these three ingredients.

Film-forming agents are just what they sound like; they cause the polish to form a film on your nails. The film-forming agent typically used in nail polish is nitrocellulose and less often, cellulose acetate butyrate. Nitrocellulose is a highly combustible substance (it's also used in making dynamite!) that holds the nail polish ingredients together on the nail. On its own, nitrocellulose is hard and brittle, which is why it's necessary to add plasticizers.

The plasticizers keep the film on your nails flexible, which helps the polish adhere and prevents chipping. Some examples of plasticizers are acetyl tributyl citrate, camphor, and formaldehyde resin.

Some common nail polish ingredients and their purpose:

Ingredient Name	Description
Nitrocellulose	Film Former
Cellulose Acetate Butyrate	Film Former
Butyl Acetate	Solvent
Ethyl Acetate	Solvent
Isopropyl Alcohol	Solvent
Acetyl Tributyl Citrate	Plasticizer
Stearalkonium Hectorite	Suspension Agent
Acrylates Copolymer	Film Former
Silica	Suspension Agent
Propyl Acetate	Solvent
Phthalic Anhydride	Plasticizer
Trimellitic Anhydride	Plasticizer
Adipic Acid	Plasticizer
Formaldehyde Resin/Tosylamide Resin	Plasticizer
Camphor	Plasticizer
Butylene Glycol	Solvent
Triphenyl Phosphate	Plasticizer
Stearalkonium Bentonite	Suspension Agent
Benzophenone-1	UV filter
Dibutyl Phthalate*	Plasticizer
Toluene*	Solvent
Formaldehyde (actually Methylene Glycol)*	Nail hardener (used in treatments)

* Chemicals considered part of the Big 3 and not contained in products that are advertised as 3-free.

Other Ingredients

Beyond the basic building blocks of polish, there are also substances added that give it color, add special effects, provide benefits to the nails themselves, or help with making the formula easy to apply.

Polyethylene Terephthalate (PET) is a fancy name for glitter, specifically glitter made from polyester, which is solvent-resistant to avoid color loss when added to nail polish.

Mica is used to give polish a pearly or frosty effect.

Silicones (such as dimethicone) are sometimes added to enhance the flow of the polish out of the bottle and onto the nail.

Suspension Agents such as stearalkonium hectorite or silica are what enable the color particles or glitter pieces to remain uniformly suspended in the polish. A lack of these ingredients is why adding glitter or pigment to plain clear polish results in everything sinking to the bottom of the bottle.

Titanium Dioxide is a white powder used to create pastel colors and to help with opacity.

Aluminum in powdered form is used to create chrome or metallic shades and can even be treated to create an additive that produces a holographic or color-changing effect.

Formaldehyde (a misnamed methylene glycol) is added to treatments to help harden the nails.

Oils of many different varieties can be added in small amounts to help moisturize the nails.

Mass-produced nail polish uses different types of powdered pigments for color. These are often listed in the ingredients as FD&C colors or by their CI (Color Index) name. Mixing these powdered pigments into polish requires some pretty serious equipment—and working with highly flammable ingredients—in order to get a smooth and consistent color in the finished product. For personal use, I suggest working with existing polishes as they are easily available, relatively inexpensive, safe to use, and only contain ingredients allowed for use in nail polish.

To begin mixing your own colors, it's best to start with the primaries: red, yellow, and blue, plus white and black. These should be easy to find in most drugstores, and often you will find the difference in prices reflects the concentration of the pigments used—but not always. This is where experimentation will come in! Highly pigmented colors (those that apply opaque on the nail with fewer coats) will give you more flexibility in the color/concentration of your final product, while less pigmented colors (sheer/jelly finishes or those that require multiple coats to appear opaque on the nail) will be easier to work with, particularly for beginners.

Some examples of inexpensive polish lines and colors that make good primary colors for use in mixing:

Red
Sinful Colors Ruby Ruby (jelly)
NYC New York Color Big Apple Red
Wet n Wild Wild Shine Red Red

Yellow
Sinful Colors Unicorn (pastel)
NYC New York Color Midtown Mimosa

Blue
Sally Hansen Xtreme Wear Pacific Blue
Pure Ice Strapless
Sinful Colors Endless Blue

White
Wet n Wild Wild Shine French White Crème
Sinful Colors Snow Me White
NYC New York Color French White Tip

Black
Wet n Wild Wild Shine Black Crème
Sinful Colors Black on Black

If you are trying to create a specific color, it may be possible to find something close and adjust the color slightly to get the exact hue you're aiming for.

Glitters

Glitters will add depth, dimension, and sparkle to your polish. You can really go wild with different colors and sizes of particles to create something truly unique. There are a few important things to know, however, when working with these types of ingredients.

The main consideration when working with glitters is that they should be solvent-resistant and stable in the nail polish base you are using. This means the color will not break down, change, or tint the polish; and the glitter will not bend, curl, or otherwise change shape. The majority of glitter sold in craft stores or labeled as craft glitter is *not* solvent-resistant, because it's more expensive to produce glitter with this property and isn't necessary when working with the types of materials normally used in craft-type projects. There are many online sources available where you can purchase solvent-resistant glitter for use in making your own nail polish in quantities as little as a few teaspoons at a time. Another alternative is to use an existing glitter polish—this makes things easier because you don't need to test it and you also don't need to have a special polish base to suspend the glitter.

Glitters come in many different sizes and finishes. The following is a guide to help you understand some of the more commonly used ones:

Glitter Finishes

Shiny or reflective glitter is the most common and likely what you think of when you hear the word *glitter*. This type of glitter is available in the widest range of colors and sizes.

Matte glitter is relatively new and comes in both pastel and primary colors. It does not appear shiny and is much more likely to be solvent-resistant because of the way it's manufactured. (However, there are some matte glitters—particularly neons—that may still bleed; so, it's important to be informed about and to test your glitters.) This type of glitter finish is also less likely to be seen in mass-produced polishes.

Opalescent-finish glitter flashes different colors depending upon the angle from which you're viewing it. The most common colors you will find are a red/orange and a green/blue color shift, and often both of these are mixed together for a rainbow effect.

Holographic glitter is shiny glitter with a coating that flashes the full rainbow when exposed to light. The most commonly used holographic glitters in mass-produced polishes are silver and gold, but this finish is available in different colors as well.

Glitter Sizes

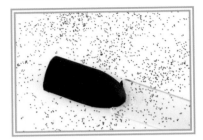

.008 inches

This is generally the smallest size of glitter that is easily available to purchase and will give you a coarse shimmery effect on the nail. This size glitter can also be used to create a full-coverage glitter polish, though the finish will dry somewhat gritty.

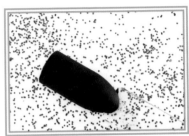

.015 inches

This size can be used in combination with .008 to give more dimension to a glitter top coat or full-coverage glitter polish.

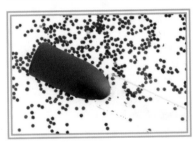

.035 inches

This is generally the largest size of glitter you will see in mass-produced polishes. It is also the size at which you may start to see curling.

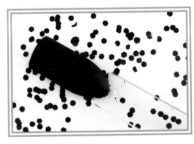

.062 inches

This glitter is large and thus more prone to curling; however, it is not so large that you won't find a good assortment of colors available. Most suppliers don't consider curling a "defect" in glitter, so it's always important to test these larger sizes if curling is something you want to avoid.

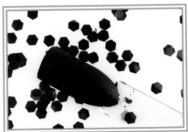

.125 inches

This is HUGE glitter! Generally, this is the largest size you will see available for sale or in nail polish and is usually in very limited colors.

Glitter Shapes

With the explosion in popularity of glitter nail polish, there have been more and varied shapes of glitter available. In addition to the traditional hexagon, square, and bar/string shapes, you can now find circles in several different sizes and finishes. There are also hearts, stars, diamonds, flowers, crescents, butterflies, bows, skull and crossbones, snowflakes, pumpkins, and other holiday-themed shapes—even Christmas trees. Commercial polish companies have yet to really take advantage of these new shapes, so this is an opportunity to make your creations unique!

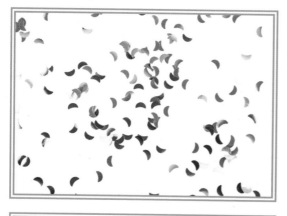
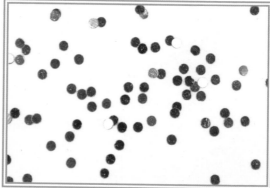
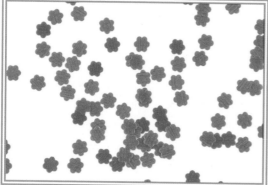
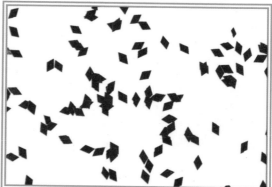

Thinners

Nail polish thinner is specifically made to be added to nail polish to replace some of the solvents that can evaporate over time. This means there is no reason ever to get rid of a polish simply due to the fact that it has thickened. You should also be careful NEVER to use acetone or nail polish remover–type products (or a thinner that contains acetone) to thin a polish, as this will eventually break down the polish and ruin it.

You will likely find having thinner on hand to be an indispensable tool to help you in your polish mixing. Many times the only thing standing in the way of a tricky-to-apply, streaky polish and an easily applied, gorgeous finish is adding a bit of thinner. Don't worry if you end up adding too much! Simply leaving the cap off for a bit and checking it periodically will get you back to your desired consistency.

Nail polish thinner often can be found in beauty supply stores—Sally Beauty Supply carries one by the Beauty Secrets brand that works very well.

Suspension Base

If you have ever tried to make your own polish by using a basic clear coat you have likely run into the issue of sinking pigments, glitter, or both. This is because clear polish doesn't contain anything to ensure that these types of additives remain suspended. In order to make sure that your polishes look as good in the bottle as they do on the nail, you will want to have some suspension base on hand—this is even more important if you will be mixing polishes using glitters and not just combining existing polishes.

Suspension base is probably not something you will be able to pick up locally in a store (yet!), but there are many options available online. How much to get depends on how much and what types of polish you plan to make. Crèmes and jellies will use the least amount and, in fact, you can mix the suspension base with plain clear most of the time. For large or chunky glitter polishes, you will want to use undiluted suspension base. For everything related to polish making, I always recommend to start small first and test, test, test. There are many different formulations of base available. They will vary with application, wear, and durability, and will react differently with different types of glitters.

If ordering online isn't an option for you, or if you are struck with the creativity bug and need to make something RIGHT NOW, there are still a few alternatives you can try. Matte top coat often contains enough suspension ingredients to support pigments and smaller glitters, and there are a few superfine glitter polishes on the market that can also be used as a base. One of my favorite combinations is using eye shadow and matte top coat together to create a shimmery matte polish. NYC makes a great inexpensive matte top coat (Matte Me Crazy), and ORLY makes two polishes (Love Each Other and Fifty-Four) that contain very fine, nearly invisible glitter that can be substituted for suspension base in a pinch.

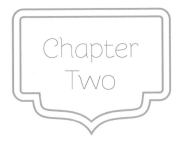

Chapter
Two

Equipment: What You'll Need and Why

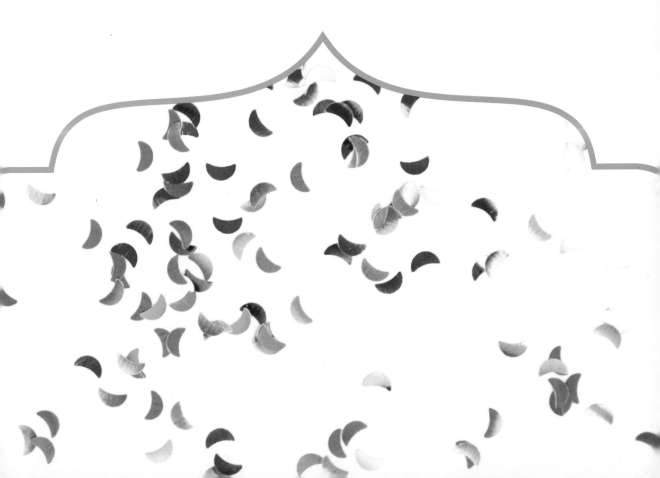

Mixing your own nail polish colors doesn't really require anything more than a bottle to mix it in, but there are definitely things you can have on hand that will make the process easier and your results more consistent. Safety is also an important consideration when working with nail polish. This chapter will cover the various pieces of equipment you can use to make your polishes and will describe what they do so you can decide for yourself how much or how little you need to start out.

What makes mixing nail polish (or applying nail polish) dangerous is the exposure to the volatile solvents that evaporate as it dries. If you are using powdered pigments, there is also an inhalation hazard from the dust. This is serious stuff! I always recommend mixing and applying nail polish in a well-ventilated area away from heat or open flames. In addition to this, I also recommend wearing a mask and gloves at a minimum. I have found that nitrile gloves are thin enough not to make working with your hands difficult and are also solvent-resistant. They can usually be found in the painting supplies section of the hardware store. Try putting on hand cream every time you wear gloves — it's great for your cuticles and nails!

For a face mask, I recommend using at least a half face mask with a replaceable vapor/particulate filter. I use the 3M P100 cartridge filter.

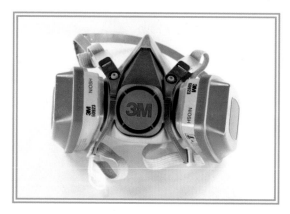

A good filter will work so well that you will not be able to smell *any* nail polish while you are working. Make sure to purchase the correct size for your face/head (most reusable masks will come in sizes small, medium, and large).

For extra safety credit, consider designating a long-sleeved shirt as your "polish mixing shirt" to protect your clothes and skin from any small spills.

Make sure also to protect your work surface! Nail polish and remover can quickly ruin the finish on almost any non-nail surface they come in contact with. In order to protect your work surface, you will want to make sure you have a nonporous covering to work on. I prefer and recommend using a silicone baking mat for this purpose for two reasons: it's flexible and can be rolled up and easily stored away when not in use; and any spills can be left to dry and simply peeled off the sheet and disposed of safely in your household trash. A glass cutting board can also be used but will require that you use acetone to clean up any spills.

Though it's possible to mix directly into the bottle, it is much easier to control the end result and make changes as you go if you mix in a separate container. You can also mix more than one bottle at a time this way. Silicone baking cups (muffin size) are ideal for mixing polish. They are inexpensive and can be reused indefinitely by simply allowing the excess nail polish to dry, and then turning the cup inside out and peeling the dried polish off.

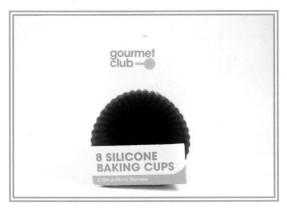
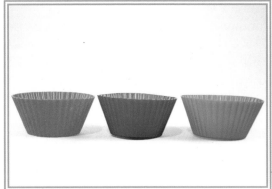

Small bathroom-size paper cups (Dixie cups) can also be used, but are one-time-use only and generate a lot more waste. You also need to work somewhat quickly as over time, the polish may eat through the paper cup.

When mixing in a cup, you will also want something to stir with. I prefer to use a long wooden cotton swab, with cotton at only one end. You can also use stirring utensils made of stainless steel or silicone, if you don't mind cleaning up with acetone after each color you make.

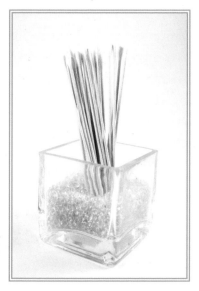
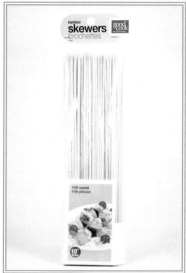

Another disposable option is wooden barbecue skewers.

If you are working with loose glitter or pigments, you will want a tiny scoop for dispensing and measuring. I have used the tiny spoons labeled "Dash/Pinch/Tad," a special plastic "glitter scoop" from a craft or scrapbooking store—or I've even cut the end off of a straw at a diagonal. The key thing to remember here is consistency. If you want to be able to re-create any of your recipes, you will want to make sure you're using the same measuring tools. For consistency, I have used the Dash/Pinch/Tad spoons along with their associated weights for the recipes that use loose glitter in this book.

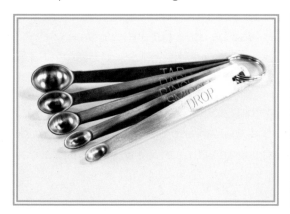
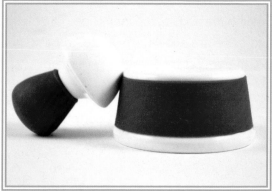

A mortar and pestle will be helpful if you intend to use a lot of eye shadows to color your polishes. One that has a pestle with a wide base will work best.

A digital jewelry or kitchen scale will be invaluable, particularly if you are mixing in cups rather than in the bottle, and for following or reproducing your recipes. You will want something that measures in .1-gram increments at a minimum and has a tare function. The tare function will allow you to measure each ingredient as you add it to the mix by resetting the scale to zero after the addition of each one.

Because the color in the bottle is not always a good indicator of the color you will see on the nail, it's a good idea to test your color as you go. You can buy specially made plastic wheels that contain 10 to 20 "nail" tips on them at beauty supply stores, or you can even reuse clear plastic packaging.

You will want to have plenty of pure acetone around for cleanup. I find it easiest to store it in a squeeze bottle. Just make sure the bottle is marked HDPE on the bottom so you know the acetone won't break down the plastic.

Bottles

As you start mixing and creating using existing polish, you will likely find that you are emptying bottles as quickly as you fill new ones. It is easy and economical to clean and reuse them.

1 Make sure the bottle is as empty as you can get it by pouring out any remaining contents onto a paper towel or paper plate. This will allow the discarded polish to dry so you can properly dispose of it. If the mixing ball is still in there, you can capture it by pouring the polish through a metal strainer; you can reuse the ball as well.

2 Add acetone to the bottle about half-way full; replace the cap, and shake, shake, shake until you can see that all the polish has been removed from the sides of the bottle.

3 Empty the acetone out and repeat step 2 if necessary. It's important to note that you shouldn't leave acetone in the bottles with the cap on for too long (such as overnight)—the acetone might eat the bristles in the brush and ruin it.

4 Using a cotton swab (Q-tip) moistened with acetone, clean the threads in the cap.

5 If there are labels on the bottle, remove them and clean up any remaining adhesive with—yes, more acetone.

6 If the bottle is printed, you can use the "foil method" to remove the ink. Unwind one cotton ball—wet it with acetone and wrap around the bottle. Cover this with aluminum foil.

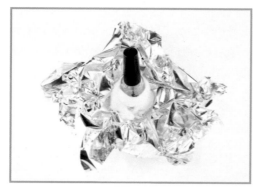

7 Press the foil around the bottle and let it sit for 10 to 20 minutes.

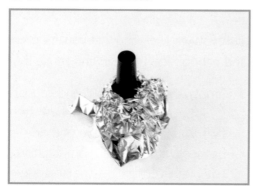

8 Unwrap the foil.

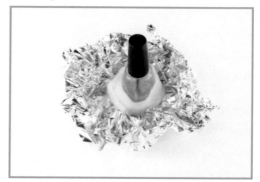

9 The lettering should just wipe off.

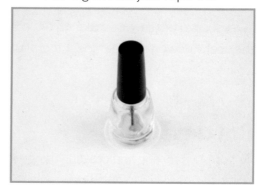

10 The final step is to let the bottle sit without the cap on for 30 minutes or so, to ensure that every last bit of acetone has evaporated out before you refill it.

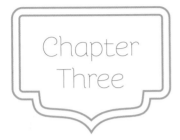

Chapter
Three

Recipes and Techniques

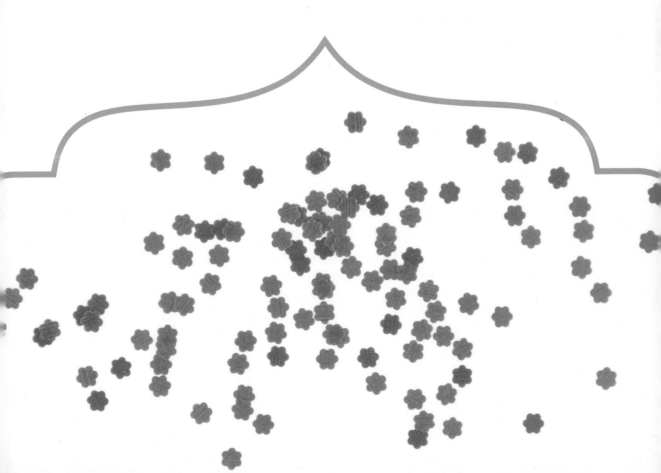

Now that you're familiar with all the components that go into making nail polish, it's time to start mixing! To get you started, there are recipes here that cover using everything from eye shadow to glitter to holographic pigments.

For each recipe where I've used a specific color polish there is a general descriptive name given and then the specific polish used is mentioned in parenthesis. Don't worry about finding the exact polish—while I've tried to use polishes that are commonly available today, companies are constantly discontinuing colors and creating new ones. Work with what you have, and can find, using these recipes as a guide.

I used a scale to document these recipes as I developed them, and so many of the quantities are listed in grams. Please note, however, that you can easily translate these weights into volumes; for nail polish, 1 gram (weight) = 1 milliliter (volume). For instance, if the recipe calls for 7 grams of polish, this is also equal to 7 milliliters, or roughly half of a full-size 15-milliliter bottle.

Pay attention as you make each recipe; you can get a feel for the consistency and color, opacity, and ratios of ingredients at each step of the process. This will help you as you go "off road" and begin to create your own recipes. Also note that I have given these recipes descriptive names, leaving you the fun part of coming up with a name.

Polishes Made with Eye Shadow

Before you get started: if you are mixing directly in the bottle, make sure to crush the eye shadow before adding to the bottle.

Also, keep in mind the packaging on many eye shadows will understate the amount of shadow by weight. For example, the packaging for the shadow used in the Purple Matte Shimmer recipe states there is .8 grams of shadow—but after measuring, there is actually twice that amount. Always measure! These polishes will dry with a matte finish. Try adding a shiny top coat to change the look, or try some of the nail art techniques to mix matte and shiny finishes for contrast.

Purple Matte Shimmer

Ingredients

1.5 grams shimmery purple eye shadow (Revlon Diamond Lust in Plum Galaxy)

1–2 grams thinner

11 grams matte top coat (NYC New York Color Matte Me Crazy)

4 grams superfine glitter polish (ORLY Love Each Other)

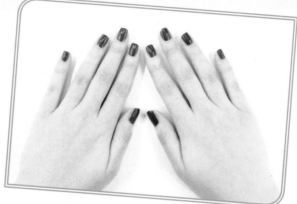

Instructions

1 Break up the eye shadow as much as possible, using a mixing stick to remove it from the packaging.

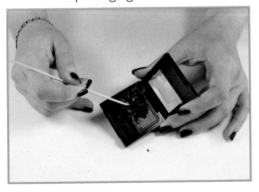

2 Measure out the eye shadow, making sure to crush it up as much as you can so you have a smooth powder.

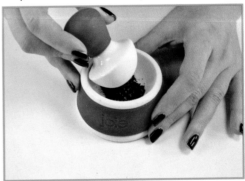

3 Add the eye shadow to your mixing container.

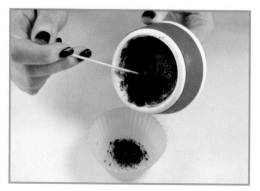

4 Add the thinner, which will appear to melt the eye shadow on contact.

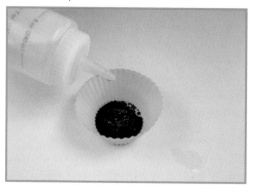

5 Mix well until there are no lumps—this is very important for a good formula!

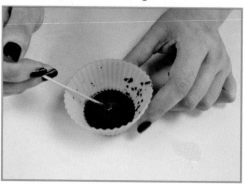

6 Now add in your matte and glitter polishes and mix again.

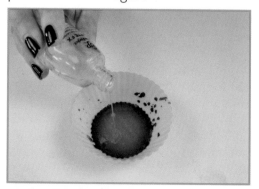

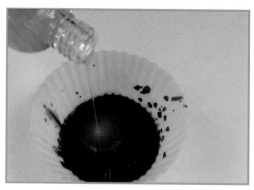

7 Finally, pour the finished polish into the bottle.

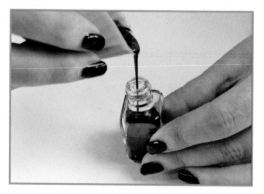

8 Now add a brush and cap.

Blackened Silver

Ingredients

1.5 grams shimmery silver eye shadow (Revlon Diamond Lust in Celestial Silver)

1–2 grams thinner

1 bottle matte top coat (NYC New York Color Matte Me Crazy)

2 grams black polish (Wet n Wild Black)

2 grams clear or suspension base (can also substitute matte top coat or fine glitter polish)

Instructions

1 Measure out the eye shadow and add it to your mixing container, making sure to crush it up as much as you can so you have a smooth powder.

2 Add the thinner, which will appear to melt the eye shadow on contact.

3 Mix well until there are no lumps—this is very important for a good formula!

4 Finally, add in your matte and black polishes and suspension base, and mix well

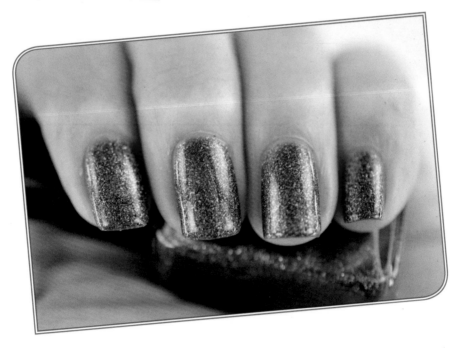

Red with Gold Shimmer

Ingredients

2 grams gold sparkly eye shadow

2 grams thinner

3.5 grams red polish (Sinful Colors Ruby Ruby)

10 grams suspension base (can also substitute matte top coat or fine glitter polish)

Instructions

1 Measure out the eye shadow and add it to your mixing container, making sure to crush it up as much as you can so you have a smooth powder.

2 Add the thinner, which will appear to melt the eye shadow on contact.

3 Mix well until there are no lumps.

4 Finally, add in your red polish and suspension base, and mix well.

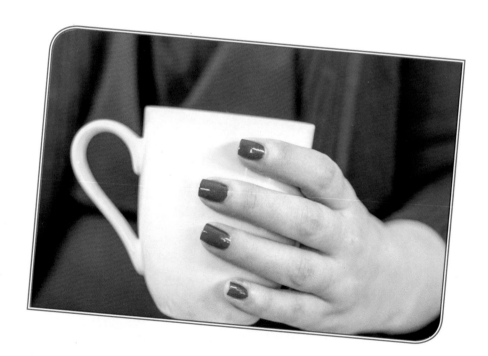

Purple with Pink Shimmer

Ingredients

4 grams purple matte eye shadow (no sparkle)

2 grams thinner

10 grams pink sparkle nail polish (FingerPaints Sparkle Top Coat)

Instructions

1 Measure out the eye shadow and add it to your mixing container, making sure to crush it up as much as you can so you have a smooth powder.

2 Add the thinner, which will appear to melt the eye shadow on contact.

3 Mix well until there are no lumps.

4 Finally, add in your pink sparkle nail polish, and mix well.

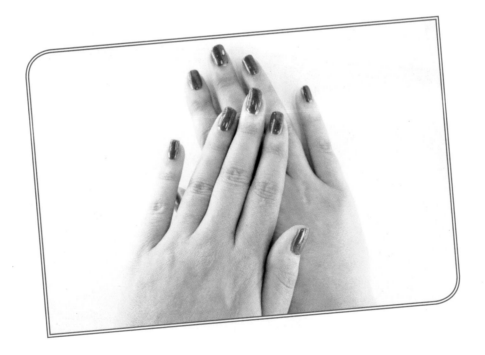

Silver Sparkly Top Coat

Ingredients

1.5 grams shimmery silver eye shadow (Revlon Diamond Lust in Celestial Silver)

1–2 grams thinner

1 gram .008 silver holographic glitter (Wet n Wild Fantasy Makers Confetti in Silver)

15 grams suspension base (can also substitute matte top coat or fine glitter polish)

Instructions

1 Measure out the eye shadow and add it to your mixing container, making sure to crush it up as much as you can so you have a smooth powder.

2 Add the thinner, which will appear to melt the eye shadow on contact. Start with one gram and add a second if needed to dissolve completely.

3 Mix well until there are no lumps.

4 Finally, add in your glitter and suspension base, and mix well.

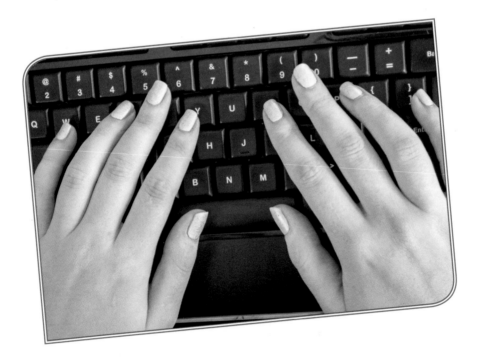

Tan Shimmer

Ingredients

4 grams tan or off-white eye shadow

1–2 grams thinner

2 grams white polish (Wet n Wild Wild Shine French White Tip)

11 grams suspension base (can also substitute matte top coat or fine glitter polish)

Instructions

1 Measure out the eye shadow and add it to your mixing container, making sure to crush it up as much as you can so you have a smooth powder.

2 Add the thinner, which will appear to melt the eye shadow on contact. Start with 1 gram and add a second if needed to dissolve completely.

3 Mix well until there are no lumps.

4 Finally, add in your white polish and suspension base, and mix well.

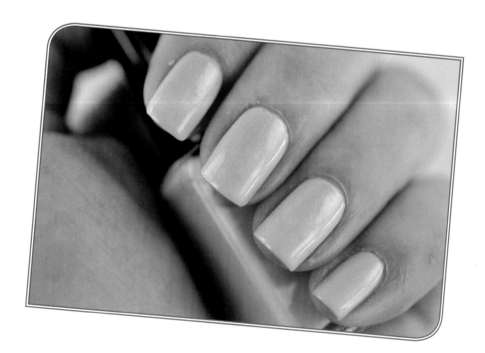

Olive Shimmer

Ingredients

1 gram gold shimmer shadow (Wet n Wild Fantasy Makers Confetti in Gold)

2–3 drops thinner

5 grams black polish (Wet n Wild Wild Shine Black)

10 grams suspension base (can also substitute matte top coat or fine glitter polish)

Instructions

1 Measure out the eye shadow and add it to your mixing container, making sure to crush it up as much as you can so you have a smooth powder.

2 Add the thinner, which will appear to melt the eye shadow on contact. Start with 2 grams and add a third if needed to dissolve completely.

3 Mix well until there are no lumps.

4 Finally, add in your black polish and suspension base, and mix well.

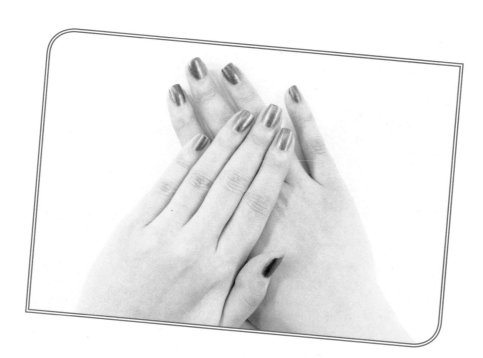

Grey with Turquoise Shimmer

Ingredients

2 grams shimmery turquoise eye shadow (L'Oreal Infallible in Dive Right In)

1 gram thinner

1 gram black polish (Wet n Wild Wild Shine Black)

2 grams white polish (Wet n Wild Wild Shine French White Tip)

10 grams suspension base (can also substitute matte top coat or fine glitter polish)

Instructions

1 Measure out the eye shadow and add it to your mixing container, making sure to crush it up as much as you can so you have a smooth powder.

2 Add the thinner, which will appear to melt the eye shadow on contact.

3 Mix well until there are no lumps.

4 Finally, add in your black and white polishes and suspension base, and mix well.

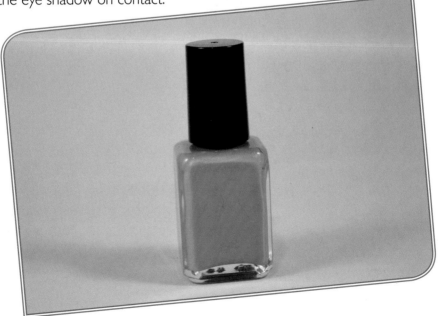

Combining Nail Polishes

If you are mixing in the bottle, add half the suspension base and then the rest of the ingredients. Finally, add the rest of the base. This will make it easier to combine ingredients when shaking.

Black with Iridescent Glitter and Shimmer

Ingredients

3 grams large iridescent glitter polish (Revlon Heavenly)

3 grams tiny iridescent glitter polish (Color Club Si Vous Please!)

1 gram turquoise shimmer polish (Sally Hansen Triple Shine Sparkling Water)

1 gram black polish (Wet n Wild Wild Shine Black)

7 grams suspension base

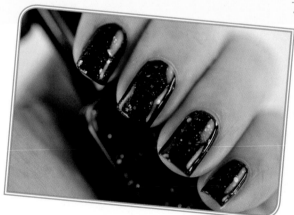

Instructions

1 Begin with your mixing container on a scale and use the tare function to reset to 0.

2 Add 3 grams of the large iridescent glitter polish.

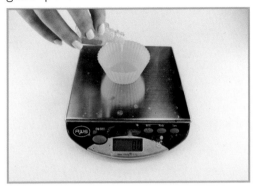

3 Tare the scale and add 3 grams of tiny iridescent glitter polish.

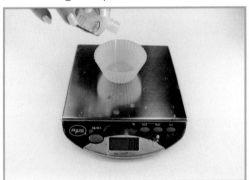

4 Tare the scale and add 1 gram of turquoise shimmer polish.

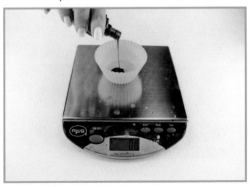

5 Tare the scale and add 1 gram of black polish.

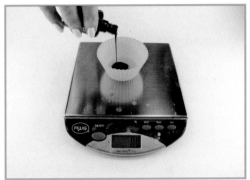

6 Tare the scale one last time and add 7 grams of suspension base.

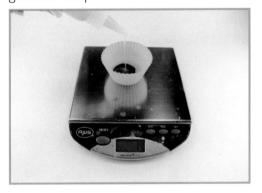

7. Mix everything together thoroughly

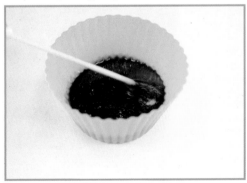

Mermaid Shimmer Polish

Ingredients

1 gram magenta glitter polish (Sally Hansen Diamond Strength Wedding Crasher)

1.5 grams yellow polish (NYC New York Color Midtown Mimosa)

1 gram blue polish (NYC New York Color Boat Basin)

1 gram turquoise shimmer polish (Jesse's Girl Confetti)

1 gram blue shimmer polish (Pure Ice Déjà vu)

1 gram blue glitter polish (ORLY Stone Cold)

1 gram blue shimmer polish (Bongo Sweet Cheeks)

1 gram blue glitter polish (Pure Ice Strapless)

6g suspension base

Instructions

Combine the above ingredients and mix well.

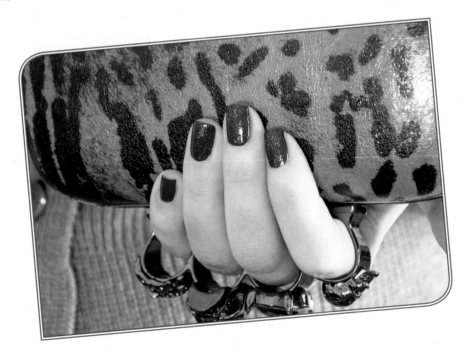

White Base with Blue and Pink Glitter

Ingredients

10 grams suspension base

2.5 grams white polish (Wet n Wild Wild Shine French White Crème)

2 grams blue glitter (Pure Ice Strapless)

2 grams fuchsia glitter (Sally Hansen Xtreme Wear Pinky Ring)

Instructions

Combine the above ingredients and mix well.

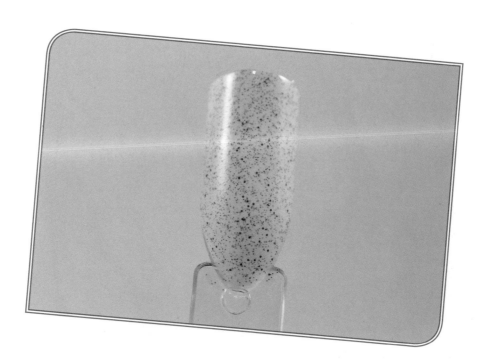

Pink with Iridescent Glitter and Shimmer

Ingredients

6 grams suspension base

1 gram white polish (Wet n Wild Wild Shine French White Crème)

2 grams large iridescent glitter polish (Sally Hansen Complete Salon Manicure Snow Globe)

2 grams tiny iridescent glitter polish (Color Club Si Vous Please! or Blue Cross Snowman)

4 grams blue shimmer polish (Bongo Sweet Cheeks)

Instructions

Combine the above ingredients and mix well.

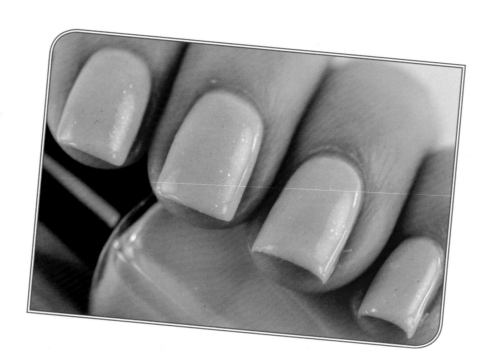

Blue with Glitter

Ingredients

8 grams suspension base

.5 gram white polish (Wet n Wild Wild Shine French White Crème)

6 grams mixed glitter polish (NYC New York Color Starry Silver Glitter)

.5 gram blue shimmer polish (Pure Ice Déjà vu)

1 gram blue polish (Sally Hansen Xtreme Wear Pacific Blue)

Instructions

Combine the above ingredients and mix well.

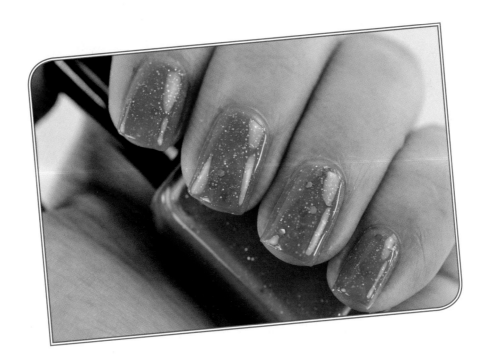

Blue with Copper

Ingredients

8 grams suspension base

6 grams copper glitter polish (Sally Hansen Complete Salon Manicure in Copper Penny)

2 grams slate blue polish (L.A. Girl Color Pop Deep Sea)

Instructions

Combine the above ingredients and mix well.

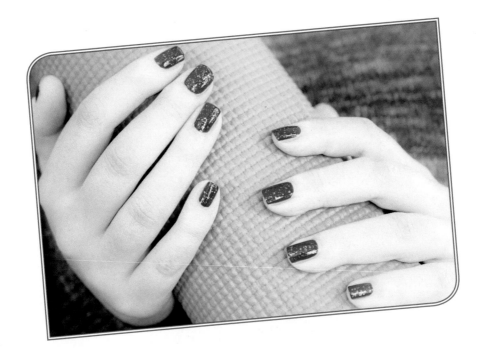

Yellow Party Glitter

Ingredients

12 grams suspension base

2 grams mixed rainbow glitter polish
(Pure Ice It's Complicated)

.5 gram yellow polish (NYC New York
Color Midtown Mimosa)

.5 gram white polish (Wet n Wild Wild
Shine French White Crème)

Instructions

Combine the above ingredients and mix
well.

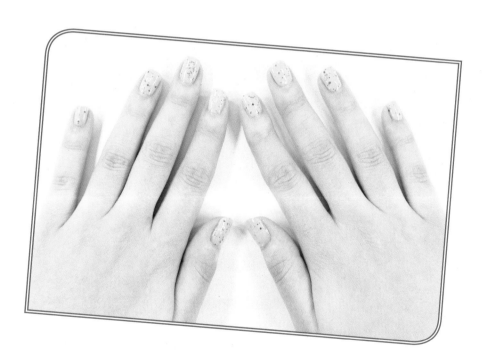

Loose Glitter and Glitter Mixes

1 drop = .1 gram

1 pinch = .2 gram

1 dash = .3 gram

1 tad = .7 gram

Blue with Fuchsia Glitter

Ingredients

12 grams suspension base

3 grams blue polish (NYC New York Color Boat Basin)

.4 gram (2 pinches) .015 fuchsia metallic hex glitter

.4 gram (2 pinches) .035 fuchsia metallic square glitter

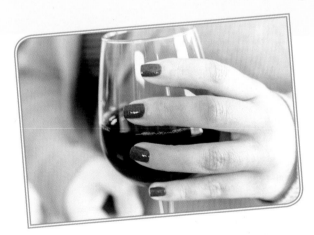

Instructions

1 Add the suspension base and blue polish to a mixing cup.

2 Then add in each glitter, measuring level spoonfuls.

3 Mix and pour into a 15-milliliter bottle.

4 Now SHAKE, SHAKE, SHAKE to combine everything.

Alternatively, if you are mixing in a bottle:

1 First add just enough suspension base to cover the bottom of the bottle.

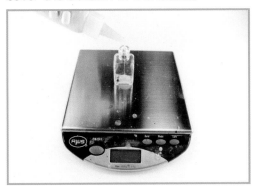

2 Using a scale, add the 3 grams of blue polish.

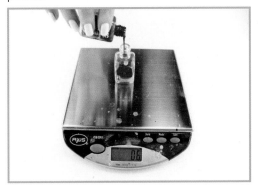

3 Using a paper funnel, measure and add the glitters.

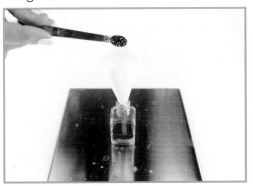

4 Add suspension base to the shoulder of the bottle.

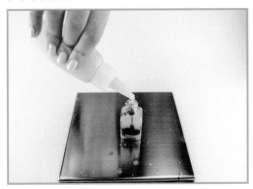

5 Add a brush and a cap.

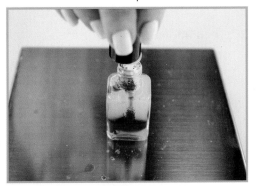

6 Shake to mix.

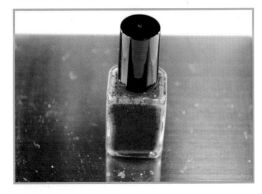

Fuchsia with Blue Glitter

Ingredients

13 grams suspension base

2 grams hot pink polish (Sinful Colors Feeling Great)

.4 gram (2 pinches) .015 blue metallic hex glitter

.4 gram (2 pinches) .035 blue metallic hex glitter

Instructions

1 Add the suspension base and the hot pink color polish to a mixing cup.

2 Then add in each glitter, measuring level spoonfuls.

3 Mix and pour into a 15-milliliter bottle. (Alternatively, if you are mixing in a bottle, fill it about half full with suspension base and then add the color polish. Next add the glitters using a paper funnel and top off with more base.)

4 Shake to mix.

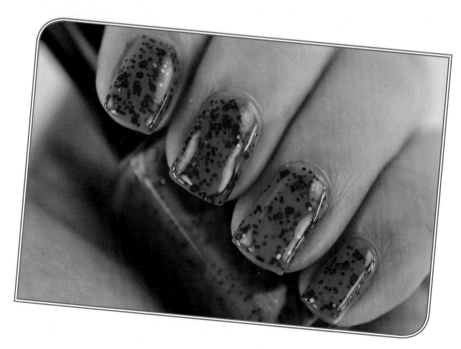

Galaxy in a Bottle

Ingredients

9 grams suspension base

2 grams deep navy polish (Color Club Blue-topia)

1.5 grams blue shimmer polish (Bongo Sweet Cheeks)

1 gram pink shimmer polish (Nail Pops Pink Shimmer)

.5 gram holographic glitter polish (China Glaze Fairy Dust)

1 gram gold and pink glitter polish (Sinful Colors Gilded)

1 drop (.1 gram) .015 matte white hex glitter

1 drop (.1 gram) .035 matte white hex glitter

1 drop (.1 gram) .035 green metallic hex glitter

Instructions

1 Add the suspension base and the polishes to a mixing cup.

2 Then add in each glitter, measuring level spoonfuls.

3 Mix and pour into a 15-milliliter bottle. (Alternatively, if you are mixing in a bottle, fill it first with the color polishes. Then add the glitters using a paper funnel, and top off with suspension base.)

4 Shake to mix.

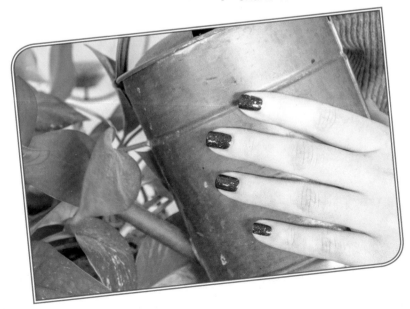

Black and White Glitter with Holographic Sparkle

Ingredients

14 grams suspension base

1 gram holographic concentrate

.2 gram (1 pinch) .015 matte white hex glitter

.2 gram (1 pinch) .015 matte black hex glitter

.2 gram (1 pinch) .035 matte white hex glitter

.2 gram (1 pinch) .035 matte black hex glitter

Instructions

1 Add the suspension base and holographic concentrate to a mixing cup.

2 Then add in each glitter, measuring level spoonfuls.

3 Mix and pour into a 15-milliliter bottle. (Alternatively, if you are mixing in a bottle, fill it about half full with suspension base, then add the holographic concentrate. Next add the glitters using a paper funnel, and top off with more base.)

4 Shake to mix.

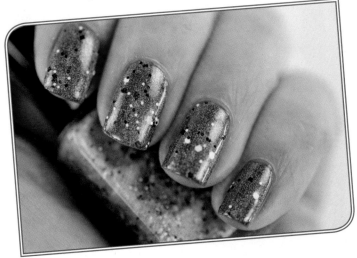

Green and Gold Full-Coverage Glitter

Ingredients

15 grams suspension base

.7 gram (1 tad) .008 gold metallic hex glitter

.7 gram (1 tad) .008 green metallic hex glitter

.7 gram (1 tad) .008 green to gold shift iridescent hex glitter

Instructions

1 Add the suspension base to a mixing cup.

2 Then add in each glitter, measuring level spoonfuls.

3 Mix and pour into a 15-milliliter bottle. (Alternatively, if you are mixing in a bottle, fill it about half full with suspension base. Then add the glitters using a paper funnel and top off with more base.)

4 Shake to mix.

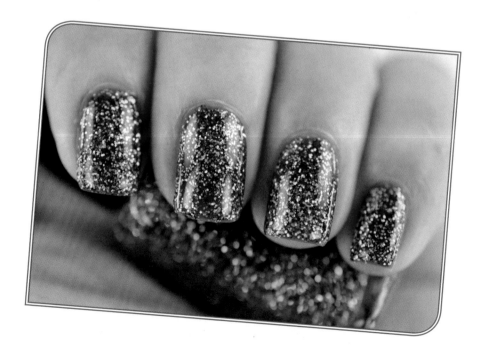

Matte Full-Coverage Glitter – Mixed Sizes

Ingredients

15 grams suspension base

.7 gram (1 tad) .015 lavender matte square glitter

.7 gram (1 tad) .008 grey matte glitter

.7 gram (1 tad) .008 light yellow matte glitter

Instructions

1 Add the suspension base to a mixing cup.

2 Then add in each glitter, measuring level spoonfuls.

3 Mix and pour into a 15-milliliter bottle. (Alternatively, if you are mixing in a bottle, fill it about half full with suspension base. Then add the glitters using a paper funnel and top off with more base.)

4 Shake to mix.

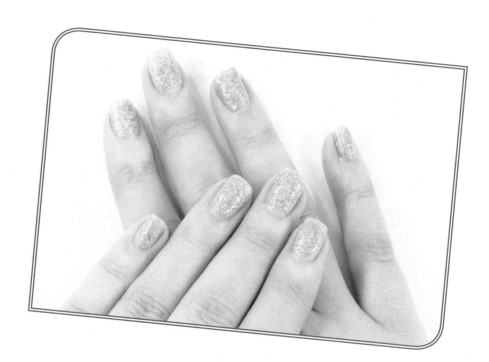

Matte Full-Coverage Glitter – Sunset

Ingredients

15 grams suspension base

.7 gram (1 tad) .008 peach matte glitter

.7 gram (1 tad) .008 watermelon matte glitter

.7 gram (1 tad) .008 light yellow matte glitter

Instructions

1 Add the suspension base to a mixing cup.

2 Then add in each glitter, measuring level spoonfuls.

3 Mix and pour into a 15-milliliter bottle. (Alternatively, if you are mixing in a bottle, fill it about half full with suspension base. Then add the glitters using a paper funnel and top off with more base.)

4 Shake to mix.

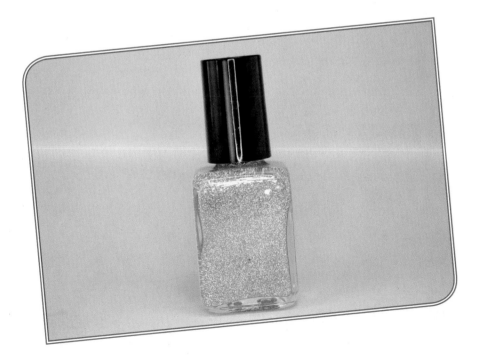

Inspired by a Picture Top Coat

Inspiration for your handmade polishes can come from anywhere—here, I am showing how a perfume sample card inspired me. The pink flowers are represented by the pink flower glitter, the brown bar glitters represent the branches, and the green and white glitters represent the leaves and highlights.

Ingredients

15 grams suspension base

.2 gram (1 pinch) .125 brown metallic bar glitter

.6 gram (2 dashes) matte light pink flower-shaped glitter

.2 gram (1 pinch) .025 matte green hex glitter

.2 gram (1 pinch) .015 matte white hex glitter

Instructions

1 Add the suspension base to a mixing cup.

2 Then add in each glitter, measuring level spoonfuls.

3 Mix and pour into a 15-milliliter bottle. (Alternatively, if you are mixing in a bottle, fill it about half full with suspension base. Then add the glitters using a paper funnel and top off with more base.)

4 Shake to mix..

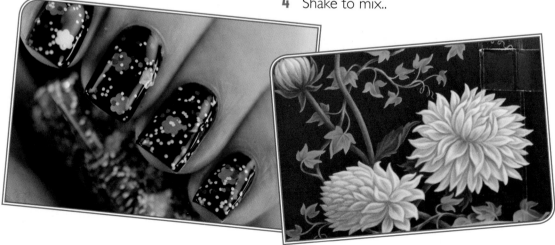

Matte Rainbow Glitter Top Coat

Ingredients

15 grams suspension base

1.5 grams rainbow glitter mix (Glitter Unique All Mixed Up!)

Instructions

1 Add the suspension base to a mixing cup.

2 Then add in the glitter mix.

3 Mix and pour into a 15-milliliter bottle. (Alternatively, if you are mixing in a bottle, fill it about half full with suspension base. Then add the glitter using a paper funnel and top off with more base.)

4 Shake to mix.

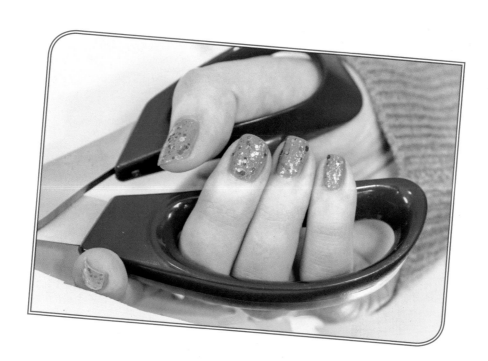

Pastel Glitter in a Creamy Base

Ingredients

12 grams suspension base

3 grams off-white shimmer polish
(Wet n Wild Megalast Break the Ice)

.7 gram (1 tad) matte pastel glitter mix
(Glitter Unique Pastel Glitter Mix)

Instructions

1 Add the suspension base and off-white shimmer polish to a mixing cup.

2 Then add in the glitter mix, measuring level spoonfuls.

3 Mix and pour into a 15-milliliter bottle. (Alternatively, if you are mixing in a bottle, fill it first with the color polish. Next add the glitter using a paper funnel and top off with suspension base.)

4 Shake to mix.

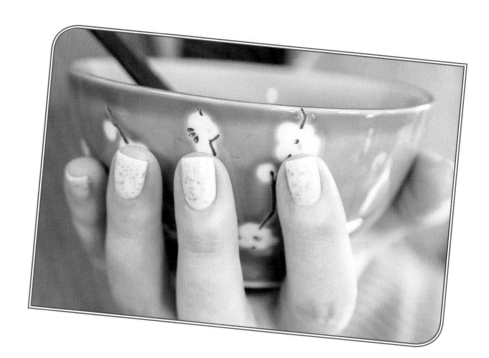

Special Effects Additives

Colorshift with Flakies

This recipe uses a special pigment that goes by the trade name ChromaFlair. It produces a brilliant shift of color when viewed at different angles. ChromaFlair is available for purchase online premixed into nail polish base. For the most intense color shift, apply over a coat of dark polish (such as black, dark purple, or navy).

Ingredients

11 grams suspension base

3 grams ChromaFlair blue/red (1 gram pigment dispersed in 15 milliliters of polish)

2 grams red/orange flakie polish (Essie Shine of the Times)

Instructions

1 Add the suspension base and Chroma-Flair to a mixing cup.

2 Then add in the flakie polish.

3 Mix and pour into a 15-milliliter bottle. (Alternatively, if you are mixing in a bottle, fill it first with the ChromaFlair and the flakie polish. Next, top off with suspension base.)

4 Shake to mix.

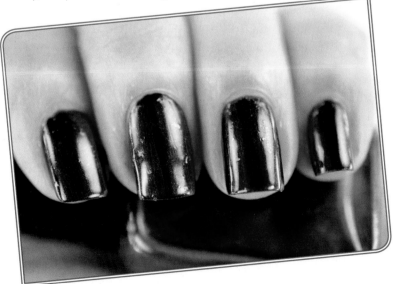

Holographic Polishes

Holographic polishes were once hard to find and in very limited supply—but recently they've become more popular. Due to the cost of the pigments to make them, they can be quite expensive. But you can easily make your own using "holographic concentrate," which you can find online. The recipes that follow were all made using a concentrate made from 1 gram of holographic powder in 15 grams of suspension base.

When creating polishes using holographic pigment, it's important to understand that currently all available pigments are silver in color, which means they will "grey out" anything you add them to, depending upon the concentration. It can be a delicate balancing act to get the right amount of rainbow sparkle (or "flame") and color concentration.

Holographic Top Coat

This can be worn over any polish to give it a holographic rainbow sparkle without greying out the base color too much.

Ingredients

15 grams suspension base

1 gram holographic concentrate

Instructions

Combine the above ingredients and mix well, taking care to add the holographic concentrate in the "middle" if you are mixing in the bottle (i.e., add 7 grams of suspension base, add 1 gram of holographic concentrate, then add the rest of the base). This will make it easier to combine ingredients when shaking.

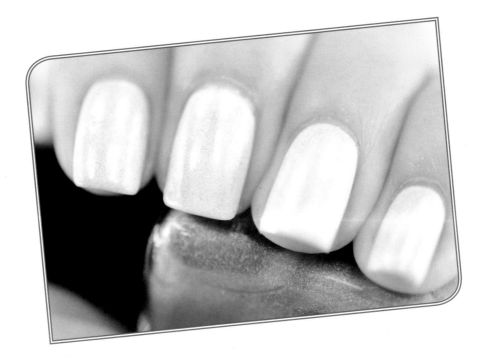

Black Holographic Polish

Ingredients

13 grams suspension base

1 gram holographic concentrate

1 gram black polish (Wet n Wild Black)

Instructions

Combine the above ingredients and mix well, taking care to add the holographic concentrate in the "middle" if you are mixing in the bottle (i.e. add 7 grams of suspension base, add 1 gram of holographic concentrate, 1 gram of black polish, then add the rest of the base). This will make it easier to combine ingredients when shaking.

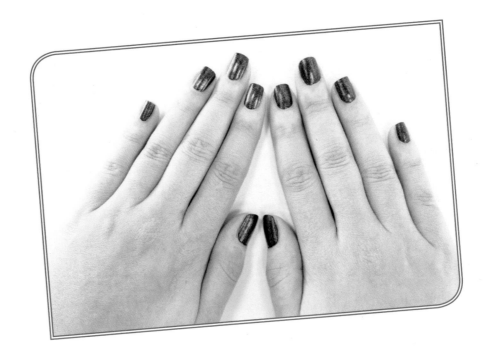

Neon Yellow Holographic Polish

The holographic effect in this is very muted, which in my experience seems to be common when combining neon pigments with holographic powder.

Ingredients

2 grams suspension base

1 gram holographic concentrate

1 bottle (12g) neon yellow polish (Wet n Wild Werewolf Vision)

Instructions

Combine the above ingredients and mix well, taking care to add the holographic concentrate in the "middle" if you are mixing in the bottle (i.e., add 7 grams of yellow polish, add 1 gram of holographic concentrate, then add the rest of the yellow and the suspension base). This will make it easier to combine ingredients when shaking.

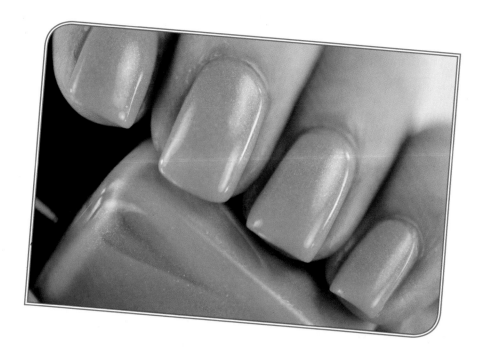

Jellies

Jelly finish refers to polishes that are more translucent than crèmes, requiring several coats to be fully opaque. They also tend to dry to a shiny finish (even without a top coat) and have an almost squishy appearance (sort of like Jell-O) on the nail. Jelly-finish polishes are a great way to experiment with layering to create different nail art effects and are easy to create using solid color polish and a clear top coat.

Several precise recipes follow for mixing jelly finish polishes, but there are a few helpful guidelines you can follow for mixing your own jellies. The first is to always begin with clear polish and add color to it a little bit at a time until you are happy with the result. Second, try to avoid using quick-dry top coats as your clear, as these will often dry too quickly to give a smooth finish. Finally, be aware there are some polishes that do not "jellify" when added to clear, such as metallic or frosty finishes.

Creamy Orange Jelly

Ingredients

11 grams suspension base (clear non-quick-dry polish can also be used)

4 grams red polish (Sinful Colors Ruby Ruby)

1 gram pastel yellow polish (Pure Ice Show Stopper)

Instructions

1 Add the suspension base and color polishes to a mixing cup.

2 Mix and pour into a 15-milliliter bottle. (Alternatively, if you are mixing in a bottle, fill it first with the color polishes and top off with suspension base.)

3 Shake to mix.

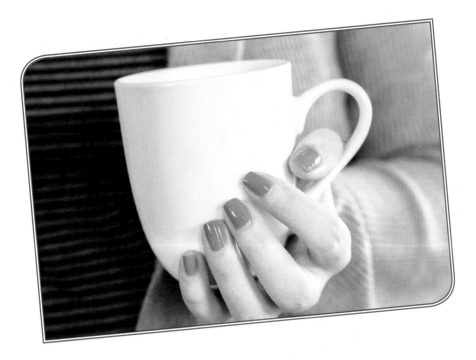

Dusty Green Jelly

Ingredients

8 grams suspension base (clear non-quick-dry polish can also be used)

1 gram blue polish (NYC Color Boat Basin)

6 grams yellow polish (NYC Color Midtown Mimosa)

1 gram dark slate-blue polish (L.A. Girl Deep Sea)

Instructions

1 Add the suspension base and color polishes to a mixing cup.

2 Mix and pour into a 15-milliliter bottle. (Alternatively, if you are mixing in a bottle, fill it first with the color polishes and top off with suspension base.)

3 Shake to mix.

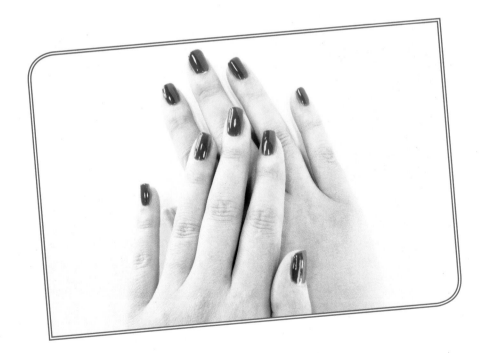

Coral Jelly

Ingredients

12 grams suspension base (clear non-quick-dry polish can also be used)

1 gram pink-based red polish (Wet n Wild Wild Shine Red Red)

5 grams yellow polish (NYC Color Midtown Mimosa)

Instructions

1 Add the suspension base and color polishes to a mixing cup.

2 Mix and pour into a 15-milliliter bottle. (Alternatively, if you are mixing in a bottle, fill it first with the color polishes and top off with suspension base.)

3 Shake to mix.

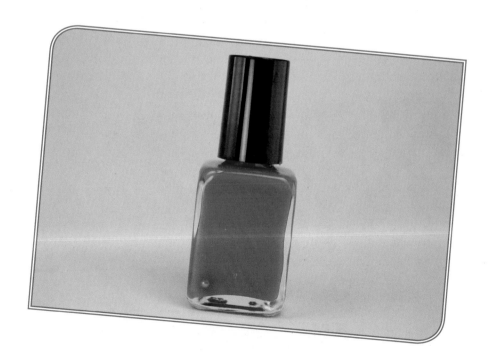

Purple Jelly

When mixing colors, red plus blue does not always equal purple. Most of my experiments mixing purple this way have turned out to be a muddy brownish color. The secret to getting a nice true purple is to mix using turquoise and magenta.

Ingredients

12 grams suspension base (clear non-quick-dry polish can also be used)

2 grams magenta polish (Sinful Colors Feeling Great)

2 grams turquoise polish (Sinful Colors Why Not)

Instructions

1 Add the suspension base and color polishes to a mixing cup.

2 Mix and pour into a 15-milliliter bottle. (Alternatively, if you are mixing in a bottle, fill it first with the color polishes and top off with suspension base.)

3 Shake to mix.

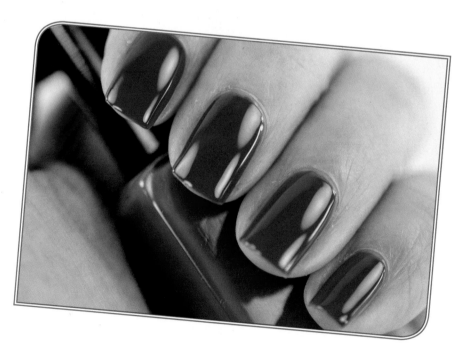

Teal Jelly

Ingredients

12 grams suspension base (clear, non-quick-dry polish can also be used)

2 grams blue polish (NYC New York Color Boat Basin)

2 grams green polish (Sally Hansen Insta-Dri I-rush-Luck)

Instructions

1   Add the suspension base and color polishes to a mixing cup.

2   Mix and pour into a 15-milliliter bottle. (Alternatively, if you are mixing in a bottle,

fill it first with the color polishes and top off with suspension base.)

3   Shake to mix.

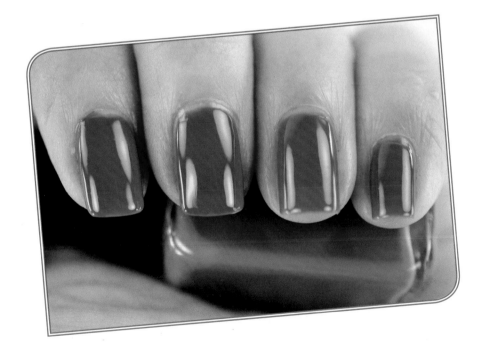

Deconstructing Nail Polish

Sometimes you will have a polish that looks amazing in the bottle but on the nail just falls flat. Here are a few suggestions on things you can do to improve the formula.

Fixing a Lumpy, Too-Opaque Glitter

Ingredients

glitter polish in a colored base

15 grams suspension base

2-3 drops thinner

solid-color polish that matches the base of the original (Wet n Wild Black, per example below)

1–2 empty polish bottles

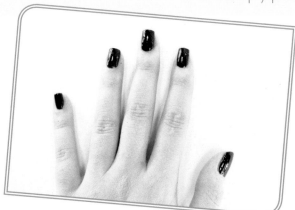

Instructions

In this case, let's say we have a polish that contains too much glitter and too much colored base, so the end result on the nail looks like an opaque lumpy mess with the added bonus of a very difficult application. What we want to do in this case is reduce the concentration of glitter first, and then add back a bit of color if necessary. The upside here is that when finished, we will end up with two bottles of improved polish.

1 First pour out the original bottle of polish into a mixing cup, taking note of the weight (the contents of most .5-ounce/15-milliliter bottles will weigh 15 grams).

2 Now you will add an equal amount of suspension base and a few drops of thinner, and mix well.

3 Test this mix on a nail wheel or piece of clear plastic to get a feel for the opacity.

If it is too sheer, now is the time to add in some of the solid-color polish. (Be careful with this step and add only a drop at a time!)

4 Mix well, and test after each drop is added until you are happy with the result.

NOTE: If you are mixing in the bottle, you will want to pour out half into a new bottle and add half of each ingredient to each bottle.

"Harvesting" Glitter from Existing Polish

So what do you do when you've found the perfect glitter, but it's in an existing polish that you can't incorporate into your design? Maybe the glitter mix itself is perfect but the clear base it's in smells so strong that you're unable to use it? Or you've got a glitter polish in a colored base that is too opaque, and adding clear will cause the final polish to be too sparse with glitter. Or maybe you love a glittery crackle polish but wish it didn't crack?

One possible solution to all of these problems is to harvest the glitter and reuse it. This is easier to do than it may seem.

Harvesting

You will need the following supplies on hand:

A solvent-safe container that is at least twice the volume of the polish you want to harvest the glitter from. For most full-size polishes, this means you need a 1-ounce container or larger. I prefer to use silicone muffin cups.

Plenty of thinner—as much as the original volume of your polish might be needed.

Something to remove/separate the unwanted polish from the glitter—either an eyedropper or some sort of straining material.

Instruction

1 Begin by emptying the polish into your container.

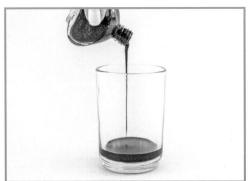

2 Now begin adding thinner, mixing it in thoroughly as you go. What you are trying to do is thin the polish to the point where the ingredients, which are suspending the glitter, become so diluted that the glitter sinks to the bottom.

3 Keep adding thinner a bit at a time.

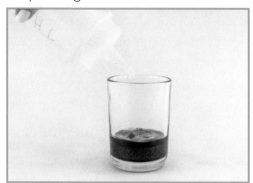

4 Continue mixing until this happens.

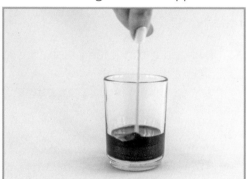

5 Once all the glitter has sunk to the bottom, you are ready to remove the unwanted polish/thinner mixture.

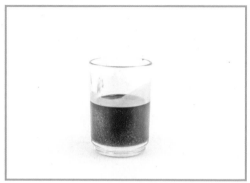

6 Use an eyedropper to carefully skim the liquid off of the top, until only the glitter is left. This will leave you with a container full of glitter, ready to be mixed into your next creation!

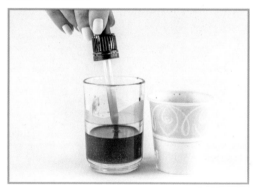

Straining Glitter

Another approach is to strain the liquid off. To do this, you will need a solvent-resistant strainer with holes small enough to catch the glitter. I have successfully used a metal mesh strainer for larger glitters; and for smaller ones, a nylon straining net commonly found at brewing supply stores (they are very large, so you will get lots of use out of one). This is another opportunity for experimentation — see what you have around the house that may work!

In this example, I am de-crackling a polish. Crackle polish is a topcoat polish that is applied over another, contrasting color. When the crackle polish dries it "cracks," leaving gaps that allow the first color applied to show through. There's no way to prevent a crackle polish from cracking, so if you like the glitter but want it to apply without cracking, you can follow these steps to remake the polish without this property.

1 The first step is to add back the suspension base.

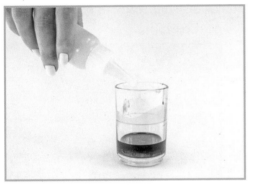

2 Mix well.

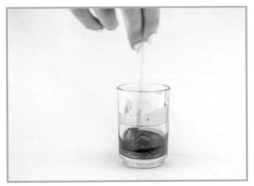

3 Next add a dark blue polish to give the color of the original.

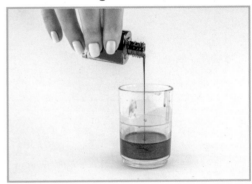

4 Pour the polish into a bottle.

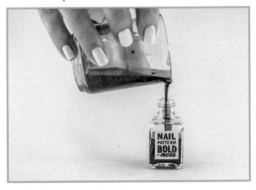

NOTE: Make sure to do this type of work in a VERY well ventilated area—and always properly dispose of the unwanted polish/thinner mixture when you're finished.

Naming and Labeling Your Creations

Nail polish is known for having fun, creative, and sometimes even bizarre names. A big part of the fun of creating your own polishes can be naming them. Of course, once you have a name, you'll want to add it to your bottles in a way that looks professional. You can do that using nothing more than a printer, adhesive labels, and some laminating film.

I prefer to use the full sheet (8½" × 11"), fully opaque white labels, but any labels with permanent adhesive (not the repositionable type) will do. Choose a fun font and print it out using either an ink-jet or laser printer. You can even hand write them; just be sure to use permanent marker.

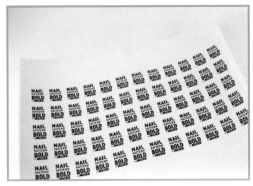

Once you've got your full sheet of labels prepared, you will want to add a layer over them to protect the labels from smudging and moisture. This is where the laminating film comes in. Full-sheet self-adhesive laminating film (Avery makes one) works well for this—you just peel off the paper backing and stick it on the printed side of your labels, smoothing as you go to eliminate air bubbles. If you aren't preparing an entire sheet—for instance, if you're just making one label for the color name—you can also substitute clear packing tape.

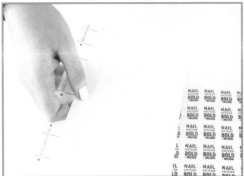

The final step is cutting out your labels. For this, you can use scissors, a paper cutter, or even scrapbooking punches.

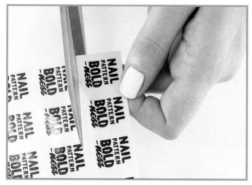

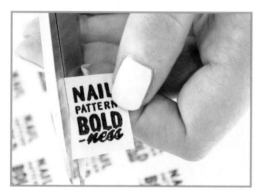

Now you're ready to put the finishing touches on your polishes! Just peel the backing off of the label and stick it on your bottle.

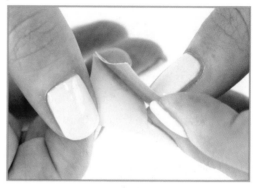

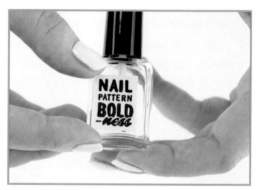

Nail Polish Application Tips and Tricks

Now that you've created a polish or two, you want to show it off in the best light possible. It is easy to do a professional-looking manicure yourself with a little practice and some helpful tips.

Why Base Coat Is Important

Base coat is an essential first step in a manicure for several reasons. All base coats are designed to help polish adhere to the nail better and most will at least reduce, if not altogether prevent, staining. Apart from these basic properties, there are many different varieties of base coats available that will have added features such as moisturizing, ridge-filling, or nail-hardening properties. Take the time to try different formulations and find the one that works best for you—you may find it makes all the difference in your final manicure!

Cuticle Flooding

The single biggest secret to a neat and professional-looking manicure is to avoid flooding the cuticle line with polish. Your goal when applying polish should be to get as close as you possibly can to this line without touching it—this includes all the layers of your manicure from base coat to color to top coat. This will take some practice, but the results are worth it! And for those times when you do get too close, the next tip will help.

Clean-Up Brush and Acetone

After you apply your color polish and before you add top coat, you can use a small brush dipped in acetone to clean up the cuticle line and any place where you may have gotten too close. Eyeliner or concealer brushes work well for this and don't have to be expensive to be effective. As you get more practice applying polish, you may find that this step becomes unnecessary.

Quick-Dry Top Coat

Quick-dry top coat does just what it sounds like—it quickly dries all the layers of polish. If you have struggled with smudging your manicures before they are dry, you need to try this. Unlike UV or LED light-cured polishes (which react with light instead of drying via evaporation like paint), it won't be rock-hard. But normally, about a minute after application, your nails will be dry enough to the touch that most smudges can be avoided. You will still need to allow a full 20 minutes or so for your polish to completely dry.

Sandwiching for Streaky Polishes

Some polishes, particularly sheers and pastels, tend to apply streaky. You can sometimes prevent this by applying an additional layer of base coat after the first coat of color polish (that is, base coat + color + base coat + color + top coat).

Foil Method for Removing Glitters

Glitter polishes are fun to wear but less fun to remove. The quickest way to remove these types of polishes (if you haven't used a peel-off base coat) is to apply an acetone-soaked piece of cotton to each nail and cover with foil, letting it sit for 5 to 10 minutes before removing. This will make easy work of even the most stubborn glitter manicures. An alternative to foil (which can quickly become wasteful if you wear a lot of glitter) is to use silicone finger grippers, usually found in an office supply store.

Peel-off Base Coat

Another way to avoid the hassle of glitter polish removal is to use a base coat that will allow you to peel off the polish instead of using acetone. An easy way to do this is to add white glue (such as Elmer's School Glue) to an empty nail polish bottle along with a few drops of water to make the consistency easier to apply. You will need to wait until the glue is completely dry (it will be clear on the nail) before you apply polish, and avoid getting your hands wet while you're wearing a manicure with this type of base coat. If the DIY route is not for you, there are also peel off base coats available for purchase. The ones that contain polyvinyl acetate are essentially the same as white glue and will appear white in the bottle. There is also a solvent-based peel-off base coat available that is quicker-drying and doesn't require avoiding water while in use; it appears clear in the bottle.

Chapter
Four

Nail Art Ideas Using Handmade Polishes

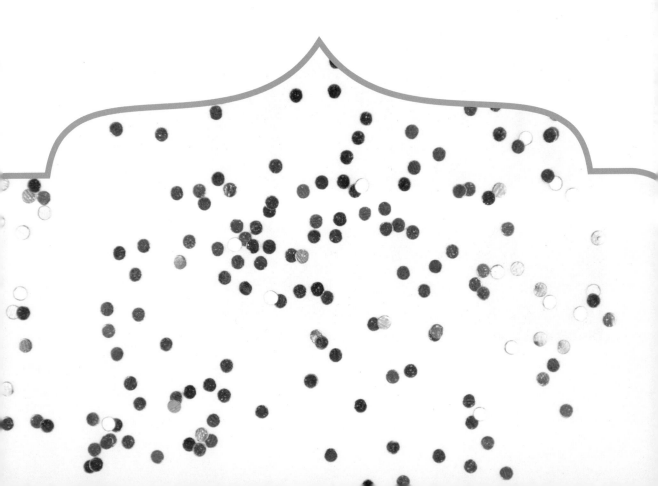

One of the advantages to mixing your own nail polish is that you can plan out some fun nail art designs using the polishes you've made. Here are just a few suggestions of looks you can try. If you've never done any nail art before and are nervous about making a mistake, try practicing these on a manicure you're about to remove first, to get a feel for the techniques.

Positive and Negative Space Using an Accent Nail

This example of nail art uses two of the recipes from this book in an accent nail manicure (a manicure in which one or more nails are painted differently from the rest of the hand).

I designed these polishes to represent the concept of positive and negative space, and you can do the same with any combination of colors. This is probably one of the easiest forms of nail art, since most of the work was done when you made the polish. It simply involves painting your accent nail (in this case I used the ring finger) with one color (the blue with fuchsia glitter) and the rest of the nails with the "opposite" color (the fuchsia with blue glitter).

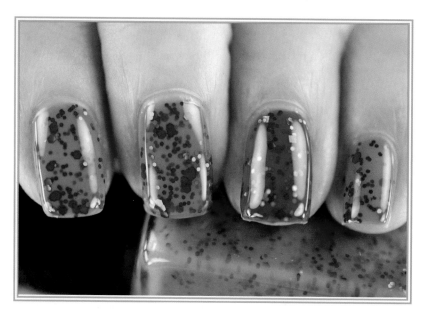

Jelly Sandwich

A "jelly sandwich" manicure refers to a method of painting your nails in which a layer of glitter is sandwiched in between layers of sheer polish. Because of the sheerness of the jelly polish the glitter shows through, giving the final manicure some depth and subtly changing the colors of the glitter as they are seen through the tint of the polish.

For this manicure, I started with two coats of Coral Jelly polish (recipe on page 65). You don't need to be concerned about any visible nail line at this point because the additional layers of polish will conceal it.

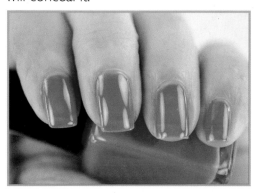

Next I applied one layer of the black and white glitter top coat with holographic shimmer.

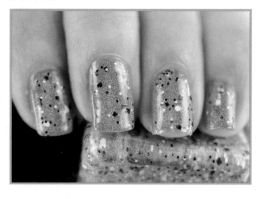

Finally, I finished with another coat of Coral Jelly and then a quick-dry top coat.

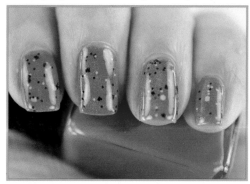

Decals (Lisa Pavelka brand)

You can find lots of material for nail art at the craft store—I found these water-slide decals in the jewelry section. They are perfect for nail art because of their small size.

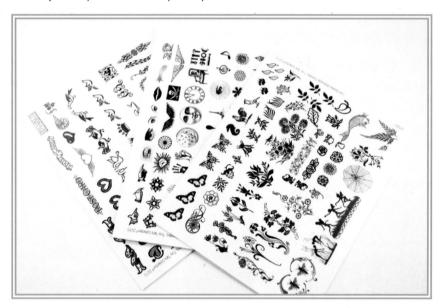

The first step is to paint your nails with a fun background color. For this manicure, I used one coat of white polish followed by one coat of the Silvery Sparkly Top Coat. Once your polish is dry to the touch, you are ready to begin applying decals.

1 Cut out each decal as close to the design as possible—this will help you get a smooth finish on the nail.

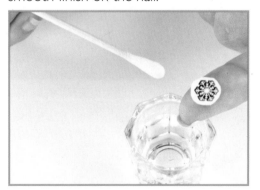

2 Next apply a few drops of water to the back of the decal and wait a minute or so for the water to absorb into the backing paper and loosen the decal.

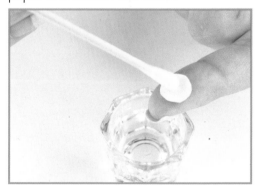

3 Now place the decal on your nail and smooth it down before applying a generous layer of top coat to seal the decal on.

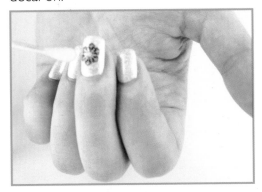

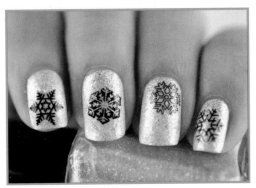

Creating Tape Stencils Using Scrapbooking Punches

There are lots of fun designs available as paper punches that can be used to create stencils for nail art.

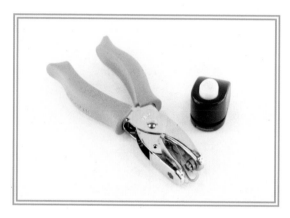

1 The trickiest part for me was figuring out how to get a clean punch in a piece of tape. What I found works well is to put a piece of masking tape onto some leftover sticker paper backing—I used the backing from a sheet of laminating film for this example.

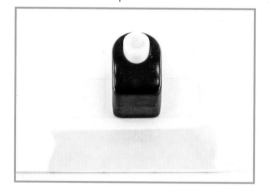

2 Now you can easily punch your design into the tape and paper combo.

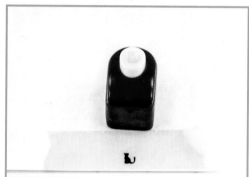

3 Place the tape onto your nail and press down FIRMLY to ensure a good seal; otherwise, your polish will bleed into the edges and you won't get a crisp image.

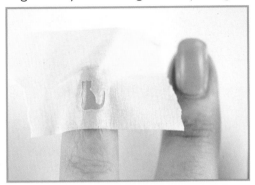

4 Now paint a layer of polish over the stencil.

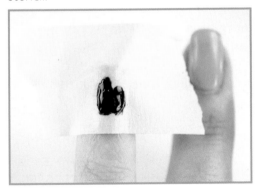

5 Let it sit for just a bit (maybe 30 seconds) and then remove the tape while the polish is still wet. After the tape is removed, let it dry for another minute or so before applying top coat to avoid streaking.

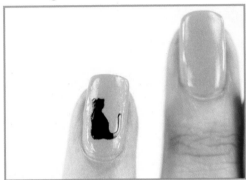

Galaxy Nails

I love the look of galaxy nails, which is why I wrote the recipe for Galaxy in a Bottle (recipe page 49). The only thing it's missing is the *nebula* (the colorful cloud), which can be added using a few eye shadow applicator sponges.

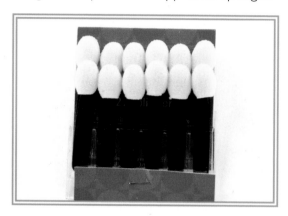

I used white, pink, and light green polishes for this, but any lighter opaque colors should work. In addition to the sponge applicators, you'll want to have a palette to work on—I used a piece of cardstock.

Begin by painting your nails with two to three coats of Galaxy in a Bottle. Once they are dry to the touch, you can begin sponging your colors on.

1   Add a few drops of the color you are working with to your palette and load up your sponge, blotting if necessary before you start on the nail.

2   I began with white, then did green, pink, and white again for depth, going in a somewhat diagonal direction on each nail.

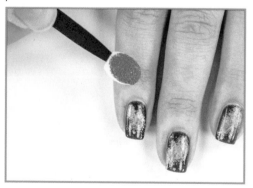

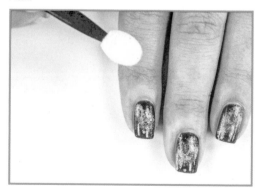

3 Once you are happy with your sponging, add one thin coat of Galaxy in a Bottle to tie everything together and give it depth. You want to make sure you apply as thin a coat as possible; otherwise, you will cover up most of the color you just added.

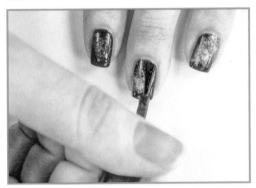

4 The last step is to apply a generous coat of top coat.

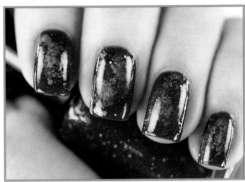

Gel Pens

Gel pens work very well to draw designs directly onto the nail. And until they are sealed with top coat, the nail can be wiped off—making it easy to start over if you make a mistake. For this manicure, I used gel pens in neon colors (Gelly Roll pens) to create a striped pattern on each nail.

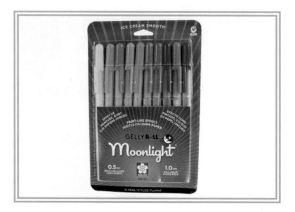

1   Start by applying your base color. Add a matte top coat before you begin drawing with the gel pens. This provides a nice surface for the gel ink to grip onto.

2   Once the matte top coat is dry you can begin drawing your designs. I stuck to something simple and just drew straight lines in different directions on each nail, beginning with pink and continuing through the colors of the rainbow.

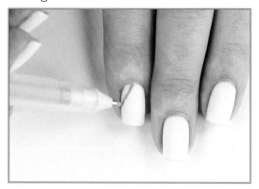

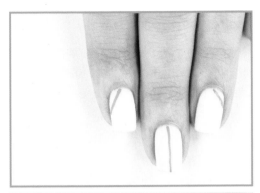

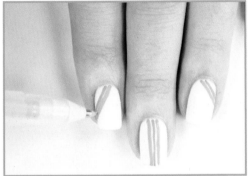

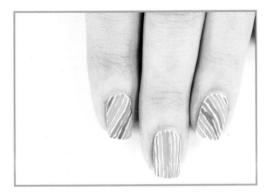

3 When you are finished drawing, seal the design with top coat.

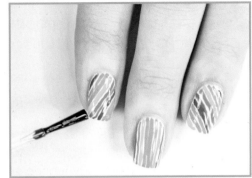

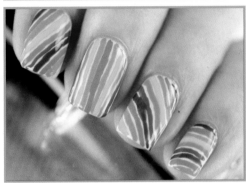

Glitter Gradient Using Makeup Sponge

A glitter gradient is a type of nail art technique where glitter is applied to the nail with heavier coverage at the tips, tapering to nothing as you get closer to the cuticle line. Alternatively, you can concentrate coverage at the cuticle line and taper toward the free edge.

For this manicure you will need a wedge makeup sponge, a palette, and a glitter polish. I am using the Green and Gold Full-Coverage Glitter recipe (see page 51) for this example.

1 Begin by painting your nails with a base color and wait for it to dry to the touch. Once your nails are ready for the glitter, pour some out onto your palette and pick it up using the makeup sponge.

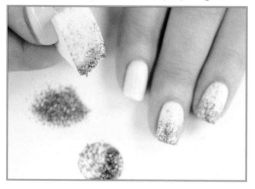

2 Now begin blotting the sponge onto your nail, touching the middle section of your nail only a few times and then concentrating on the tip.

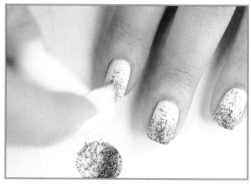

3 When you are satisfied with the amount of glitter on each nail, seal with top coat.

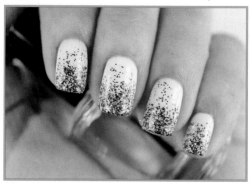

Cutting up Nail Polish Strips

Nail polish strips, a recent development, allow you to "paint" your nails quickly with no drying time, and they come in all different kinds of fun designs. The strips are available as stickers, which are peeled off to remove, and also as actual polish (in a sticker-like format), which is removed using polish remover. Either type will work for this method. All you will need are some nail polish strips and a pair of scissors.

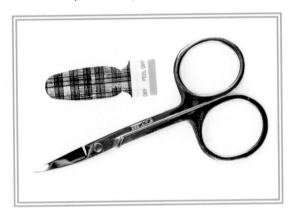

You will begin by painting your nails with a base color and letting it dry. This technique can also be used to quickly freshen up a manicure that has chipped along the free edge.

1 Using the scissors, cut a design in the nail strip, keeping in mind that you want to cut from the side opposite the tab, which allows you to easily peel the strip from its backing.

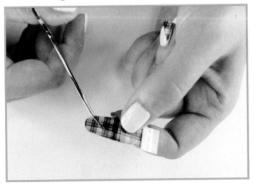

2 Now remove the backing and place the decal on your nail.

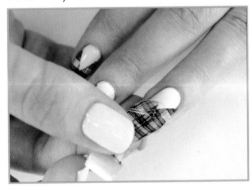

3 Once you have it in position, press down firmly to smooth it out. File the free edge to remove any excess nail strip.

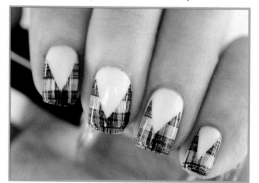

Dot Method (Bobby Pin)

You can buy a special tool to create dots on your nails but a bobby pin or toothpick works just as well. I also like to use a palette since the size of the dots will "grow" as you go, making it necessary to blot. It's also easier to just dip your tool into a bit of polish.

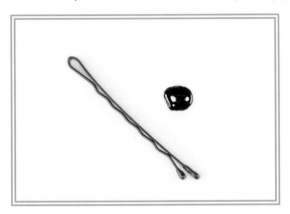

1 To start, place a few drops of polish on your palette and make sure your base polish has dried to the touch. Now just dip your tool into the polish, making a test dot on your palette to get a feel for the size. Once you're comfortable you can start adding dots to your nails in any pattern you like.

2 When finished make sure to seal with top coat.

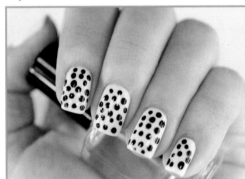

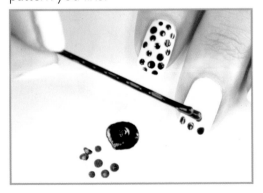

Using Loose Glitter

Instead of creating a glitter polish you can also apply loose glitter directly to the nail. This is one way to use up glitter that is not stable in nail polish. You will need a small container to hold the glitter. I used a bathroom-size paper cup—just cut the top off.

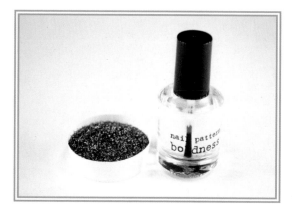

The key to this effect is dipping your nail into glitter while you have wet polish on the nail—so do each nail one at a time.

1 First apply a layer of top coat.

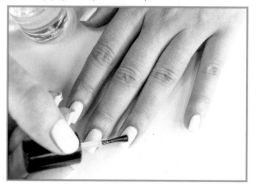

2 Then quickly dip your finger into the dish of loose glitter.

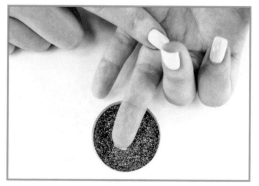

3 You will end up with some excess glitter on your fingernail.

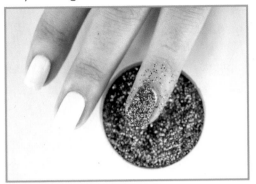

You can continue in this way for all the nails, or you can just do one as an accent nail as shown.

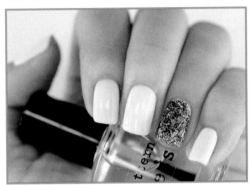

4 So blow gently to remove it before applying a final layer of top coat.

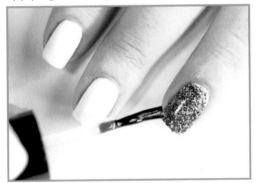

Resources

Ingredients

www.nailpatternboldness.com
Bottles, suspension base, glitters, and holographic pigment are all available here—readers of this book can use the code for 10% off all polish making supplies and kits.

www.glitterunique.com
Glitter Unique is a great resource for solvent-resistant glitter. I used their All Mixed Up! mix for Matte Rainbow Glitter Top Coat (page 55) and their Misfits on 8th Pastel Glitter mix for Pastel Glitter in a Creamy Base (page 56). The full-coverage glitter recipes also use glitter purchased here. There's a huge assortment of sizes, shapes, and colors of glitter, all available in sample-sized bags that are plenty for making one or two bottles of polish.

www.etsy.com
Etsy is another option for supplies—there are several sellers that offer suspension base, bottles, glitter, and other polish-making ingredients.

www.sallybeauty.com
The exclusive distributor of the FingerPaints brand, Sally Beauty Supply is a good source for acetone, nail wheels, and thinner. They also carry various sizes of squeeze bottles (many made from HDPE), which are great for storing acetone or mixing larger amounts of polish.

spectraflair4u.storenvy.com
Spectraflair4u is an online source for Chromaflair pigment mixed into nail polish.

Most chain drugstores carry several brands of inexpensive polish. Another way to find stores is to go to the brand's website and use the store locator; some brands will even have the option to purchase directly from their website (like L.A. Colors).

Wet n Wild (www.wnwbeauty.com)

Sinful Colors (www.sinfulcolors.com)

NYC New York Color (www.newyorkcolor.com)

L.A. Colors (www.lacolors.com)

Sally Hansen (www.sallyhansen.com)

Pure Ice—Carried exclusively at Walmart (www.walmart.com)

Orly—Available at Sally Beauty Supply (www.sallybeauty.com) or www.orlybeauty.com

FingerPaints—Carried exclusively at Sally Beauty Supply (www.sallybeauty.com)

Color Club (www.shopcolorclub.com)

Bongo—Carried at Kmart (www.kmart.com) and Sears (www.sears.com)

Jessie's Girl—carried exclusively at Rite Aid (www.riteaid.com)

Equipment

Bed Bath and Beyond carries silicone muffin cups and baking mats, glass cutting boards, and digital kitchen scales.

Hardware stores (like Lowe's and Home Depot) are a great place to find face masks and nitrile gloves.

Amazon.com is another great option—they have everything and you can usually get free shipping, too.

Nail Art Inspiration

anotherbottleofpolish.blogspot.com
Another Bottle of Polish?! is a great blog that has some really original and unique designs using Gelly pens and decals.

lavishlayerings.blogspot.com
Jenny, of Lavish Layerings, shows how simply layering polishes can give you gorgeous effects.

www.thepolishedmommy.com
The Polished Mommy is a really gifted artist, luckily she also has tons of tutorials (how-tos) to walk the rest of us step by step through some of her designs.

www.thedigitaldozen.com
The Digital Dozen is a collection of 12 bloggers that all do great nail art designs, from stamping to layering to freehand art and more.

loodieloodieloodie.blogspot.com
Loodie is a fantastic resource for learning more about nail care. Read through the archived posts to get guidance on everything from nail shape and how to file properly, to fixing a break, to choosing the right basecoat for your specific nail type.

Acknowledgments

I wish to personally thank the following people for their contributions to this book:

- Max, for his limitless patience and support, awesome photography skillz, and keeping everyone on The Schedule

- Tiger Lily, for being born with such perfect timing and providing me with the maternity leave that allowed me to finish this book

- Heather, for always encouraging me to think big

- Mimi, of Makeup Withdrawal, for her incredibly thorough feedback from day one

- Gini, of Sassy Paints, for her friendship, support, and encouragement

- Mish, of Accio Lacquer, for continuing to inspire me with her enthusiasm for all things nails, and for being one of my earliest and biggest fans

- Billy Gaeckle, for the conversation that day in the river while washing wild onions, which led to everything

- Isaac Wasuck, of wasuckphoto.com, for generously sharing his expertise

- Leah Ann Larowe, of llarowe.com, for recognizing my great ideas early on and helping me reach a wider audience than I ever could have on my own

- Kelly, my editor at Ulysses Press, for her feedback and patience with me as a first-time author

About the Author

Allison Rose Spiekermann is a patent-holding IT Architect and the founder and creative director of Nail Pattern Boldness, an independent nail polish company that specializes in unique and innovative products to help both amateur and professional nail polish enthusiasts get more out of every manicure. She is the inventor of Glitter Food, a specially designed topcoat for rough finishes, and Glitter A-Peel, a peel-off basecoat for easy removal of tenacious polishes. When she's not in the lab mixing or at her computer, she performs with and designs costumes for the electro-pop supergroup Rue Mevlana. She lives with her husband and daughter in Burlington, Vermont.